HOW TO CONTROL HIGH BLOOD PRESSURE WITH DIET

A COMPREHENSIVE GUIDE TO DIETARY ADJUSTMENTS AND LIFESTYLE CHANGES FOR EFFECTIVE HYPERTENSION MANAGEMENT

Copyright@2024

Whipkey Cramer

TABLE OF CONTENT

CHAPTER 1: UNDERSTANDING HIGH BLOOD PRESSURE..20
    CAUSES AND RISK FACTORS...................20

CHAPTER 2: THE DASH DIET AND PROVEN APPROACH 36
    WHAT IS THE DASH DIET?......................36

CHAPTER 3: ESSENTIAL NUTRIENTS FOR BLOOD PRESSURE CONTROL 45
    THE IMPACT OF SALT ON BLOOD PRESSURE 45

CHAPTER 4: FOODS TO INCLUDE AND AVOID...58
    BENEFICIAL FOODS 58

CHAPTER 5: MONITORING AND ADJUSTING YOUR DIET 74
    TRACKING YOUR PROGRESS..................74

INTRODUCTION

OVERVIEW OF HIGH BLOOD PRESSURE (HYPERTENSION)

High blood pressure, or high blood pressure, is a commonplace but extreme situation where the force of the blood towards the walls of your arteries is always too high. This accelerated stress can cause giant fitness complications, which include heart disorder, stroke, and kidney harm. Understanding the character of hypertension is critical for effective control and prevention.

Definition and Types of Hypertension:

Primary Hypertension: This is the most commonplace kind, growing step by step over many years without an identifiable motive.

Secondary Hypertension: This type is as a result of an underlying situation inclusive of kidney ailment, hormonal issues, or medicinal drug aspect consequences.

IMPORTANCE OF MANAGING BLOOD PRESSURE:

Effective management of blood stress is crucial for decreasing the hazard of heart assaults, strokes, and different cardiovascular illnesses.

By maintaining wholesome blood pressure levels, people can improve average exceptional of lifestyles and decrease healthcare expenses.

HOW DIET IMPACTS BLOOD PRESSURE

Diet plays a vital function in regulating blood stress. The meals you devour can directly have an effect on your blood pressure tiers, both undoubtedly or negatively. A balanced and nutrientwealthy eating regimen can help manage and doubtlessly lower high blood stress.

RELATIONSHIP BETWEEN DIET AND BLOOD PRESSURE:

Sodium Intake: High sodium stages can result in fluid retention and increased blood pressure.

Nutrient Balance: Consuming adequate quantities of potassium, magnesium, and calcium supports healthful blood vessel feature and enables regulate blood pressure.

Goals for Dietary Management:

Reduce Sodium Intake: Lowering sodium intake can assist save you blood pressure spikes.

Increase Nutrient Rich Foods: Incorporating meals wealthy in important nutrients can support cardiovascular health.

Promote Overall Healthy Eating Habits: Adopting a balanced diet that supports heart health can make a contribution to lengthy term blood pressure control.

IMPORTANCE OF MANAGING BLOOD PRESSURE

Managing blood pressure is vital for keeping universal fitness and well being.

1. Reducing Risk of Cardiovascular Diseases

High blood strain places greater strain on the heart and blood vessels, growing the threat of:

Heart Disease: Chronic high blood pressure can cause situations inclusive of coronary artery disorder, coronary heart failure, and coronary heart attacks.

Stroke: Elevated blood stress can purpose damage to blood vessels in the brain, growing the probability of a stroke.

2. Preventing Kidney Damage

The kidneys filter waste and extra fluid from the blood. High blood strain can harm the blood vessels in the kidneys, leading to:

Chronic Kidney Disease (CKD): Over time, CKD can development to kidney failure, requiring dialysis or a kidney transplant.

Increased Risk of Complications: Poorly managed blood pressure can exacerbate current kidney issues or cause new kidney issues.

3. Protecting Vision

High blood strain can harm the blood vessels within the eyes, doubtlessly main to:

Retinopathy: This situation reasons harm to the retina and can result in imaginative and prescient troubles or blindness if untreated.

Increased Risk of Eye Conditions: Conditions like macular degeneration or hypertensive retinopathy can broaden.

4. Enhancing Quality of Life

Proper management of blood pressure can lead to:

Improved Physical Health: Lowering blood stress can lessen the danger of great health troubles and improve universal physical properlybeing.

Better Mental Health: Managing hypertension can lessen stress and tension associated with health worries, contributing to better mental fitness.

5. Reducing Healthcare Costs

Effective control of blood stress can assist:

Decrease Medical Expenses: Preventing headaches associated with high blood stress reduces the want for luxurious treatments and hospitalizations.

Lower Long Term Costs: Maintaining suitable blood stress control can lessen the need for medicinal drugs and interventions inside the future.

6. Preventing Complications in Other Conditions

High blood stress can exacerbate different health situations, which include:

Diabetes: It can worsen blood sugar manage and growth the threat of diabetic complications.

Obesity: Hypertension and weight problems frequently pass hand in hand, and dealing with you can help enhance the opposite.

HOW DIET IMPACTS BLOOD PRESSURE

Diet performs a big position in managing and influencing blood pressure stages. The foods you consume can both make a contribution to improved blood pressure or assist hold it inside a wholesome range.

1. Sodium and Blood Pressure

Impact of Sodium:

Sodium, a key issue of table salt, is understood to raise blood strain by causing the frame to maintain water. This more fluid will increase the volume of blood in the bloodstream, setting extra strain at the walls of blood vessels.

High sodium intake is related to improved chance of growing hypertension and related complications.

Managing Sodium Intake:

Recommendations: Health organizations commonly advocate restricting sodium intake to less than 2,300 mg in line with day, with a super restrict of one,500 mg for people with excessive blood pressure or at risk.

Strategies: Reduce intake of processed and packaged ingredients, which regularly comprise excessive tiers of hidden sodium. Opt for sparkling, entire foods and use herbs and spices for flavoring in preference to salt.

2. Potassium and Blood Pressure

Role of Potassium:

Potassium helps balance sodium stages in the frame and aids in enjoyable blood vessel walls. Adequate potassium consumption can counteract the poor results of sodium and help lower blood strain.

A food regimen rich in potassium helps coronary heart fitness and overall fluid balance.

Sources of Potassium:

Foods: Include culmination like bananas, oranges, and avocados, greens which include spinach, sweet potatoes, and tomatoes, and legumes like beans and lentils.

Recommendations: Aim for a each day potassium intake of round 3,500 to 4,seven hundred mg, depending on man or woman health wishes and dietary pointers.

three. Magnesium and Blood Pressure Importance of Magnesium:

Magnesium is essential for maintaining wholesome blood stress through supporting to modify blood vessel tone and function. It additionally helps basic cardiovascular health.

Adequate magnesium intake is associated with decrease blood stress levels and a reduced threat of high blood pressure.

Sources of Magnesium:

Foods: Incorporate entire grains, nuts, seeds, leafy inexperienced greens, and legumes into your food plan.

Recommendations: The advocated each day consumption of magnesium is ready 310320 mg for ladies and 400420 mg for men, however this will range primarily based on age and health repute.

4. Calcium and Blood Pressure

Role of Calcium:

Calcium contributes to keeping wholesome blood stress through assisting right contraction and rest of blood vessel muscles. It also allows regulate blood vessel tone.

- Adequate calcium consumption can aid in preventing and handling hypertension.

Sources of Calcium:
- Foods: Include dairy products like milk, cheese, and yogurt, as well as fortified plant based totally milks, leafy vegetables, and almonds.
- Recommendations: Aim for 1,000 mg of calcium consistent with day for maximum adults, with higher desires for older adults and pregnant women.

5. Overall Dietary Patterns

The DASH Diet:

The Dietary Approaches to Stop Hypertension (DASH) diet emphasizes culmination, veggies, entire grains, lean proteins, and coffee fat dairy whilst restricting saturated fat, cholesterol, and red meats. It is designed particularly to assist decrease blood strain.

Healthy Eating Patterns:

Balanced Meals: Focus on plenty of nutrient rich meals to make sure you get a balanced consumption of essential nutrients.

Whole Foods: Choose minimally processed ingredients to avoid excessive sodium, brought sugars, and unhealthy fats.

RELATIONSHIP BETWEEN DIET AND BLOOD PRESSURE

The dating among food plan and blood strain is substantial, as the foods you devour can without delay influence your blood strain ranges.

1. Sodium and Blood Pressure

Effect of Sodium:

Sodium, frequently from salt, will increase blood strain via inflicting the frame to retain water. This more fluid will increase the quantity of blood, exerting more stress on the blood vessel walls.

High sodium consumption is strongly associated with the development and irritating of high blood pressure.

Dietary Recommendations:

Limit Sodium Intake: Aim to eat less than 2,300 mg of sodium consistent with day, with a perfect limit of one,500 mg for people with excessive blood pressure or at hazard.

Choose Low Sodium Options: Opt for fresh, whole foods over processed and packaged objects, which frequently include excessive quantities of sodium.

2. Potassium and Blood Pressure

Role of Potassium:

Potassium allows stability sodium degrees in the body and relaxes blood vessel partitions, that may help lower blood stress.

Adequate potassium consumption counteracts the results of sodium and supports usual cardiovascular fitness.

Dietary Recommendations:

Increase Potassium Rich Foods: Incorporate ingredients like bananas, oranges, candy potatoes, spinach, and beans into your food regimen.

Aim for Adequate Intake: The endorsed every day consumption is ready 3,500 to 4,seven hundred mg, relying on person wishes.

3. Magnesium and Blood Pressure

Importance of Magnesium:

Magnesium allows modify blood vessel feature and tone, which can aid in retaining wholesome blood pressure degrees.

It supports cardiovascular fitness and contributes to common blood strain regulation.

Dietary Recommendations:

Include Magnesium Rich Foods: Consume whole grains, nuts, seeds, leafy greens, and legumes.

Recommended Intake: About 310320 mg for girls and 400420 mg for men according to day.

4. Calcium and Blood Pressure

Role of Calcium:

Calcium enables preserve proper blood vessel contraction and relaxation, supporting wholesome blood pressure levels.

Adequate calcium consumption is related to lower blood strain and reduced chance of high blood pressure.

Dietary Recommendations:

Focus on Calcium Sources: Include dairy products, fortified plant based milks, leafy veggies, and almonds.

Daily Intake: Aim for 1,000 mg for most adults, with better wishes for older adults and pregnant ladies.

5. Overall Dietary Patterns

The DASH Diet:

The Dietary Approaches to Stop Hypertension (DASH) food regimen emphasizes lots of end result, vegetables, entire grains, lean proteins, and coffee fat dairy. It limits saturated fats, cholesterol, and pink meats.

This weight loss plan is designed to assist lower blood pressure and improve basic cardiovascular fitness.

Healthy Eating Patterns:

Balanced Diet: Focus on a number of nutrient rich meals to aid usual health and manipulate blood strain.

Minimize Processed Foods: Reduce consumption of processed meals high in sodium, delivered sugars, and unhealthy fat.

6. The Impact of Alcohol and Caffeine

Alcohol:

Excessive alcohol intake can enhance blood stress and contribute to hypertension. Moderation is critical—up to 1 drink in keeping with day for women and up to 2 beverages according to day for guys is commonly recommended.

Caffeine:

Caffeine can motive transient spikes in blood pressure, especially in those who are sensitive to it. While the longtime period results are debated, it is vital to display your response to caffeine and regulate intake as wanted.

7. Hydration

Importance of Adequate Hydration:

Proper hydration helps normal cardiovascular function and helps preserve healthful blood strain levels. Drinking adequate water allows regulate fluid stability and blood volume.

CHAPTER 1: UNDERSTANDING HIGH BLOOD PRESSURE

CAUSES AND RISK FACTORS

GENETIC AND LIFESTYLE FACTORS AFFECTING BLOOD PRESSURE

Both genetic and lifestyle factors play a essential function in figuring out an man or woman's blood strain stages.

GENETIC FACTORS

1. Family History:

Genetic Predisposition: Hypertension regularly runs in families. If your parents or siblings have excessive blood stress, you will be at a higher chance of developing it yourself because of shared genetic elements.

Inherited Traits: Certain genetic variations can affect how your body processes salt, manages fluid stability, and regulates blood vessel feature, all of which impact blood stress.

2. Genetic Disorders:

Primary Hypertension: While regularly multi factorial, number one hypertension may also contain genetic additives that affect blood pressure regulation.

Secondary Hypertension: Genetic conditions such as certain hormonal problems (e.G., hyperal dosteronism) can also result in expanded blood pressure.

Lifestyle Factors

1. Diet:

Sodium Intake: High intake of sodium can make a contribution to accelerated blood strain. Reducing sodium intake is essential for dealing with hypertension.

Potassium, Magnesium, and Calcium: Adequate consumption of these vitamins allows alter blood strain. Diets low in these minerals can make a contribution to higher blood strain.

2. Physical Activity:

Regular Exercise: Engaging in everyday physical interest helps decrease blood strain by way of improving heart fitness, reducing strain, and promoting healthy weight control.

Sedentary Lifestyle: Lack of bodily interest is associated with weight gain and better blood strain. Sedentary behaviors can make a contribution to high blood pressure over time.

3. Weight Management:

Obesity: Excess weight puts additional pressure on the heart and blood vessels, leading to better blood pressure. Maintaining a wholesome weight thru diet and workout can help manage and prevent high blood pressure.

Body Fat Distribution: Fat accumulation, especially around the abdomen, is related to increased blood pressure and cardiovascular risk.

4. Stress and Mental Health:

Chronic Stress: Persistent stress can lead to brief spikes in blood stress and make a contribution to the development of hypertension through the years. Managing pressure through rest techniques and mental fitness support is critical.

Mental Health Disorders: Conditions like melancholy and anxiety can have an effect on blood pressure law and normal cardiovascular fitness.

5. Alcohol Consumption:

Moderation: Excessive alcohol consumption can boost blood strain and make a contribution to hypertension. Limiting alcohol intake to moderate levels— up to one drink in keeping with day for girls and two liquids according to day for men— is suggested.

6. Smoking:

Impact on Blood Vessels: Smoking damages blood vessels, leading to expanded blood pressure and a higher threat of cardiovascular sicknesses. Quitting smoking improves blood pressure and basic heart fitness.

SYMPTOMS AND DIAGNOSIS OF HIGH BLOOD PRESSURE

High blood strain, frequently called "silent killer," might not always present considerable symptoms, specifically in its early ranges.

1. Headaches:

Persistent complications, specifically if they're severe or occur regularly, can be a signal of high blood strain.

2. Dizziness :

Feeling dizzy or lightheaded may additionally arise, particularly if blood pressure becomes very high.

3. Blurred Vision:

Elevated blood pressure can harm blood vessels in the eyes, main to vision issues.

4. Shortness of Breath:

Difficulty respiration or shortness of breath may be related to high blood pressure, specifically if it influences the coronary heart or lungs.

5. Nosebleeds:

Frequent or unexplained nosebleeds can now and again be a symptom of excessive blood pressure, although they're now not common.

6. Chest Pain:

While less common, chest ache can occur and may be related to increased blood stress affecting the heart.

7. Fatigue:

Unexplained fatigue or feeling surprisingly tired can every now and then be linked to excessive blood pressure.

It's critical to notice that many people with excessive blood strain do no longer revel in any signs. Regular monitoring is crucial for early detection and control.

DIAGNOSIS OF HIGH BLOOD PRESSURE

1. Blood Pressure Measurement:

Regular Monitoring: Blood pressure is measured the use of a sphygmomanometer (blood pressure cuff) and stethoscope, or an automatic tool. Measurements are taken in millimeters of mercury (mmHg) and recorded as systolic (top wide variety) over diastolic (bottom variety).

Diagnostic Criteria: Blood stress readings are categorized as follows:

Normal: Systolic < one hundred twenty mmHg and Diastolic < 80 mmHg

Elevated: Systolic 120129 mmHg and Diastolic < 80 mmHg

Hypertension Stage 1: Systolic 130139 mmHg or Diastolic 8089 mmHg

Hypertension Stage 2: Systolic $\geq$ 140 mmHg or Diastolic $\geq$ 90 mmHg

Hypertensive Crisis: Systolic > one hundred eighty mmHg and/or Diastolic > 120 mmHg

2. Ambulatory Blood Pressure Monitoring:

24Hour Monitoring: This test involves sporting a transportable device that measures blood stress at ordinary durations over 24 hours to assess fluctuations and affirm analysis.

3. Home Blood Pressure Monitoring:

Self Monitoring: Patients might also use a domestic blood pressure screen to music readings over the years and offer extra data for analysis and management.

4. Medical History and Physical Examination:

Assessment: A healthcare issuer will evaluate scientific records, including any signs and symptoms, own family records of hypertension, and other chance elements.

Physical Exam: The company may behavior a bodily examination to check for signs of headaches or related situations.

5. Laboratory and Diagnostic Tests:

Blood Tests: To test for underlying conditions or complications, which include kidney function and levels of cholesterol.

Urinalysis: To stumble on kidney damage or different associated troubles.

Electrocardiogram (ECG) and Echocar diogram: To investigate heart characteristic and stumble on any heart associated troubles.

HOW HIGH BLOOD PRESSURE IS DIAGNOSED

Diagnosing excessive blood stress entails several key steps to make sure accuracy and appropriate management.

1. Blood Pressure Measurement

Initial Measurement:

Technique: Blood strain is measured the usage of a sphygmomanometer (guide or computerized) and a stethoscope. The cuff is positioned across the higher arm and inflated to restriction blood waft. As the cuff deflates, the healthcare issuer listens for the sounds of blood flow to decide systolic and diastolic pressures.

Readings: Blood pressure is recorded as systolic over diastolic (e.G., a hundred thirty/eighty five mmHg).

Confirmatory Measurements:

Repeated Readings: To affirm a analysis, blood stress readings are frequently taken on more than one occasions. If the preliminary reading is high, the healthcare issuer may take additional readings at one of a kind times or visits.

2. Ambulatory Blood Pressure Monitoring (ABPM)

24Hour Monitoring:

Procedure: ABPM entails carrying a transportable blood strain display for 24 hours. The tool mechanically takes readings at everyday intervals for the duration of the day and night time.

Purpose: This technique presents a comprehensive view of blood strain styles and fluctuations over a full day, supporting to verify the diagnosis and identify capacity white coat syndrome (improved readings because of tension in a clinical setting).

3. Home Blood Pressure Monitoring

Self Monitoring:

Equipment: Patients use a home blood stress reveal to track their readings often.

Importance: Home tracking helps in detecting variations in blood stress and might help in dealing with and adjusting treatment.

4. Medical History and Physical Examination

Medical History:

Review: The healthcare company will evaluate the affected person's scientific records, such as signs, own family records of high blood pressure, and danger elements along with lifestyle behavior and current health situations.

Symptoms: Although high blood stress often has no signs and symptoms, any related signs and symptoms or health issues may be noted.

Physical Examination:

Assessment: The provider may perform a bodily exam to check for signs of complications or related fitness situations, such as swelling, heart murmurs, or signs and symptoms of organ harm.

5. Laboratory and Diagnostic Tests

Blood Tests:

Purpose: To evaluate kidney characteristic, cholesterol levels, blood sugar, and other signs that may have an effect on or be suffering from high blood stress.

Common Tests: Complete blood matter (CBC), comprehensive metabolic panel (CMP), lipid profile, and thyroid characteristic assessments.

Urinalysis:

Purpose: To check for symptoms of kidney damage or different troubles related to high blood pressure.

Analysis: The presence of proteins or blood within the urine can suggest kidney problems.

Electrocardiogram (ECG/EKG):

Purpose: To assess coronary heart feature and discover any signs and symptoms of coronary heart ailment or harm.

Procedure: Electrodes are located on the pores and skin to report the electrical hobby of the coronary heart.

COMMON SYMPTOMS AND SIGNS OF HIGH BLOOD PRESSURE

High blood strain (hypertension) is often known as the "silent killer" due to the fact it is able to now not gift important signs, particularly in its early ranges.

1. Headaches

Type: Severe headaches, often taking place behind the top.

Frequency: Persistent or frequent complications which can get worse over time.

2. Dizziness

Feeling: A sensation of spinning or unsteadiness.

Triggers: Dizziness might also arise all of sudden or in affiliation with modifications in posture or pastime.

3. Blurred or Double Vision

Vision Changes: Difficulty seeing truly or experiencing blurred imaginative and prescient.

Cause: Elevated blood pressure can harm the blood vessels within the eyes, affecting vision.

4. Shortness of Breath

Breathing Issues: Difficulty respiratory or feeling breathless, which can be associated with the strain high blood pressure puts on the coronary heart and lungs.

Activity: Shortness of breath can occur during bodily exertion or at relaxation.

5. Chest Pain

Discomfort: Pain or strain in the chest, which can also radiate to the arm, neck, or jaw.

Risk: High blood strain can make contributions to the improvement of heart sickness or angina, leading to chest pain.

6. Nosebleeds

Occurrence: Frequent or unexplained nosebleeds.

Note: While not a commonplace symptom, they are able to once in a while be associated with very high blood stress.

7. Fatigue

Tiredness: Feeling surprisingly workout or fatigued without a clear purpose.

Connection: Persistent fatigue may be associated with the impact of excessive blood stress on typical health.

8. Blood in Urine

Observation: Presence of blood within the urine, which can be seen or detected through a urinalysis.

CHAPTER 2: THE DASH DIET AND PROVEN APPROACH

WHAT IS THE DASH DIET? ORIGINS AND RESEARCH BEHIND THE DASH DIET

The Dietary Approaches to Stop Hypertension (DASH) diet turned into developed as a part of research aimed toward finding powerful dietary techniques to manipulate and decrease high blood stress (hypertension).

1. Development and Purpose

Initiation of Research:

The DASH food regimen became developed thru research funded by the National Heart, Lung, and Blood Institute (NHLBI) within the Nineties. The number one purpose changed into to analyze nutritional styles that would assist reduce blood pressure and save you hypertension.

Dietary Goals:

The DASH weight reduction plan changed into designed to emphasis foods wealthy in key vitamins regarded to impact blood strain, which include potassium, magnesium, calcium, and fiber. It additionally aimed to reduce sodium intake and restriction saturated fat and cholesterol.

2. Key Components of the DASH Diet

Nutrient Rich Foods:

Fruits and Vegetables: High in vitamins, minerals, and antioxidants.

Whole Grains: Sources of fiber and vital nutrients.

Lean Proteins: Includes rooster, fish, legumes, and nuts.

Low Fat Dairy: Provides calcium and protein while proscribing fats.

Nuts and Seeds: Rich in magnesium and healthful fat.

Reduced Sodium:

The diet emphasizes restricting sodium consumption to much less than 2,300 mg per day, with a decrease target of one,500 mg for people with excessive blood strain or at danger.

Healthy Fats:

Focus on healthful fats from sources like nuts, seeds, and olive oil, at the same time as reducing saturated fat and cholesterol from purple meats and processed foods.

3. Research and Evidence

Initial Studies:

DASH Study: The foundational studies examine, called the DASH trial, worried randomized managed trials that compared the consequences of the DASH food regimen with an average American weight loss program and a diet high in end result and vegetables. Participants following the DASH diet confirmed widespread discounts in blood pressure compared to the ones on the other diets.

Results: The DASH eating regimen reduced systolic blood strain by using approximately five6 mmHg and diastolic pressure by means of approximately 3 mmHg on common, with even greater reductions in people with better preliminary blood strain.

Long Term Research:

Follow Up Studies: Subsequent research has showed the DASH weight loss program's effectiveness in reducing blood pressure and enhancing usual cardiovascular health. Studies have shown that the weight loss program can also assist with weight management and reduce the danger of coronary heart disorder, stroke, and different continual conditions.

Variations: Research has explored versions of the DASH weight loss program, inclusive of the DASH sodium food regimen, which further restricts sodium intake and has proven additional advantages in blood stress reduction.

Clinical Guidelines:

The DASH eating regimen is extensively endorsed with the aid of foremost fitness corporations, including the American Heart Association (AHA) and the U.S. Preventive Services Task Force (USPSTF), as a key dietary approach for handling and preventing high blood pressure.

4. Broader Impact and Adoption

Public Health Recommendations:

The DASH diet has inspired nutritional suggestions and public health hints, emphasizing the importance of a balanced, nutrient wealthy weight loss plan for keeping healthful blood strain and reducing the danger of continual illnesses.

Culinary Adaptation:

The standards of the DASH eating regimen have been tailored into numerous dietary plans and meal programs, making it reachable to a broader audience and facilitating its integration into daily eating behavior.

MEAL PLANNING AND FOOD CHOICES FOR THE DASH DIET

Meal making plans at the DASH food plan involves incorporating nutrient wealthy foods that support blood pressure management at the same time as minimizing sodium, saturated fats, and brought sugars.

1. Core Principles of the DASH Diet

Focus on Nutrient Dense Foods:

Emphasize end result, greens, complete grains, lean proteins, and coffee fat dairy.

Include sources of potassium, magnesium, calcium, and fiber.

Limit Sodium and Processed Foods:

Reduce sodium intake through averting processed meals, speedy foods, and adding minimal salt in cooking.

Choose Healthy Fats:

Opt for unsaturated fat from resources like nuts, seeds, avocados, and olive oil, and limit saturated fats from red meats and complete fat dairy merchandise.

2. Daily Food Recommendations

Fruits and Vegetables:

Portions: Aim for at the least four5 servings of end result and 45 servings of greens according to day.

Examples: Fresh or frozen berries, apples, oranges, spinach, broccoli, bell peppers, carrots.

Whole Grains:

Portions: Include 6eight servings of complete grains each day.

Examples: Brown rice, quinoa, whole wheat bread, oatmeal, entire grain pasta.

Lean Proteins:

Portions: Incorporate 2 or extra servings of lean protein each day.

Examples: Skinless poultry, fish, beans, lentils, tofu, low fat dairy.

Dairy:

Portions: Consume 2three servings of low fats or fats loose dairy merchandise according to day.

Examples: Skim milk, low fats yogurt, low fat cheese.

Nuts, Seeds, and Legumes:

Portions: Include 45 servings of nuts, seeds, or legumes weekly.

Examples: Almonds, walnuts, chia seeds, flax seeds, chickpeas, black beans.

3. Sample Meal Plan

Breakfast:

Oatmeal topped with fresh berries and a sprinkle of chia seeds.

Low fat yogurt or a pitcher of skim milk.

Lunch:

Grilled fowl salad with combined veggies, cherry tomatoes, cucumber, and a vinaigrette made with olive oil and lemon juice.

A serving of quinoa or brown rice on the facet.

Snack:

A small handful of almonds or a piece of fruit (e.G., apple or banana).

Dinner:

Baked salmon with a facet of steamed broccoli and roasted sweet potatoes.

A small serving of a blended bean salad with chickpeas, bell peppers, and a light dressing.

Dessert:

Fresh fruit or a small bowl of low fats frozen yogurt.

CHAPTER 3: ESSENTIAL NUTRIENTS FOR BLOOD PRESSURE CONTROL

THE IMPACT OF SALT ON BLOOD PRESSURE

RECOMMENDED SODIUM INTAKE

Sodium is a key issue in blood pressure management, and moderating its consumption is critical for preserving healthful blood strain levels.

1. General Recommendations

For Most Adults:

Limit Intake: Aim to consume much less than 2,three hundred mg of sodium consistent with day. This advice is based totally on preferred dietary guidelines to lessen the danger of hypertension and cardiovascular ailment.

For Individuals with High Blood Pressure or Certain Health Conditions:

Ideal Intake: The American Heart Association (AHA) recommends a great restrict of one,500 mg of sodium per day. This lower limit is particularly essential for people with high blood strain, heart ailment, kidney sickness, or other situations that may be exacerbated by excessive sodium consumption.

2. Understanding Sodium Sources

Processed and Packaged Foods:

Contribution: Processed meals, including canned soups, frozen meals, and snack ingredients, frequently comprise high stages of sodium.

Advice: Check vitamins labels and choose merchandise with lower sodium content.

Restaurant and Fast Foods:

Contribution: Meals from eating places and rapid food establishments regularly incorporate high levels of sodium.

Advice: Request lower sodium options, and consider of element sizes.

Table Salt:

Contribution: Adding salt all through cooking or at the desk can extensively increase sodium consumption.

Advice: Use herbs, spices, and salt free seasoning blends to enhance taste without adding sodium.

3. Strategies to Reduce Sodium Intake

Cook at Home:

Control: Preparing meals at home allows you to govern the amount of sodium to your meals. Use sparkling substances and keep away from adding more salt.

Read Nutrition Labels:

Selection: Look for products categorized "low sodium" or "no introduced salt," and pick people with much less than a hundred and forty mg of sodium according to serving.

Use Alternative Seasonings:

Flavor: Enhance the flavor of meals with herbs, spices, lemon juice, and vinegar rather than salt.

Rinse Canned Foods:

Reduction: Rinse canned greens, beans, and different products to cast off a number of the sodium.

Potassium: How It Helps Regulate Blood Pressure

Potassium performs a crucial position in regulating blood pressure and maintaining cardiovascular fitness.

1. Balancing Sodium Levels

Fluid Balance:

Potassium helps alter fluid balance within the body by way of selling the excretion of excess sodium thru urine. High sodium stages can result in fluid retention, which increases blood extent and, therefore, blood stress.

By increasing potassium consumption, you could assist mitigate the consequences of sodium and reduce fluid retention, for that reason assisting to decrease blood stress.

Sodium Potassium Ratio:

A higher potassium intake allows counteract the poor outcomes of high sodium intake. The stability between sodium and potassium is vital for preserving ordinary blood strain stages.

2. Relaxing Blood Vessels

Vessel Dilation:

Potassium facilitates relax and widen blood vessels, which improves blood waft and decreases the strain exerted on blood vessel partitions.

This dilation impact enables to lower blood strain and improve ordinary cardiovascular feature.

3. Supporting Kidney Function

Kidney Health:

Potassium helps right kidney characteristic with the aid of assisting within the law of fluid and electrolyte stability. Healthy kidneys are critical for preserving strong blood stress levels.

By helping the kidneys filter excess sodium and fluid, potassium contributes to blood strain manipulate.

4. Reducing Blood Pressure

Clinical Evidence:

Studies have proven that growing dietary potassium intake can cause sizable discounts in both systolic and diastolic blood strain. This impact is particularly exquisite in people with high blood strain or those liable to developing high blood pressure.

The DASH (Dietary Approaches to Stop Hypertension) food regimen, which emphasizes potassium rich foods, has been proven to effectively decrease blood pressure and is broadly encouraged for hypertension management.

5. Recommended Potassium Intake

Daily Intake:

- The endorsed daily consumption of potassium for adults is approximately three,500 to 4,seven hundred mg. Specific needs may additionally vary primarily based on age, gender, and man or woman health conditions.
- It is commonly secure and beneficial for most human beings to eat potassium wealthy foods as a part of a balanced weight loss plan.

6. Sources of Potassium

Fruits:

Bananas, oranges, cantaloupe, and avocados are high quality assets of potassium.

Vegetables:

Potatoes, candy potatoes, spinach, and tomatoes are wealthy in potassium.

Legumes:

Beans, lentils, and peas are accurate assets.

MAGNESIUM AND CALCIUM: SUPPORTING HEART HEALTH

Magnesium and calcium are essential minerals that play crucial roles in retaining cardiovascular fitness, along with regulating blood strain and supporting standard heart characteristic.

1. Magnesium

Role in Blood Pressure Regulation:

Vascular Relaxation: Magnesium enables relax blood vessels by means of regulating the contraction and dilation of clean muscle cells within the blood vessel walls. This rest reduces vascular resistance and lowers blood strain.

Electrolyte Balance: It performs a function in maintaining right electrolyte stability, that's vital for everyday heart rhythm and blood strain.

Supporting Heart Function:

Heart Rhythm: Magnesium is critical for the proper functioning of the heart's electric system. It helps maintain a regular coronary heart rhythm and might save you irregular heartbeats (arrhythmias).

Preventing Cramps: Adequate magnesium ranges assist save you muscle cramps and spasms, inclusive of the ones affecting the heart.

Sources of Magnesium:

Leafy Greens: Spinach, kale.

Nuts and Seeds: Almonds, pumpkin seeds.

Whole Grains: Brown rice, quinoa.

Legumes: Black beans, lentils.

Fish: Salmon, mackerel.

2. Calcium

Role in Blood Pressure Regulation:

Vascular Contraction and Relaxation: Calcium is involved in the contraction and relaxation of blood vessels. Adequate calcium levels guide wholesome blood vessel characteristic and make contributions to maintaining ordinary blood strain.

Blood Vessel Function: Calcium helps modify the contraction of the smooth muscle cells in blood vessels, that may have an effect on blood strain.

Supporting Heart Function:

Heart Muscle Function: Calcium is important for the contraction of heart muscle groups. It guarantees the coronary heart beats efficaciously and keeps a regular rhythm.

Blood Clotting: Calcium is essential for the proper clotting of blood, which is essential for preventing immoderate bleeding and helping cardiovascular fitness.

Sources of Calcium:

Dairy Products: Milk, yogurt, cheese.

Leafy Greens: Kale, bok choy.

Fortified Foods: Fortified plantbased totally milks (e.G., almond, soy) and cereals.

Fish with Bones: Sardines, salmon.

IMPORTANCE OF MAGNESIUM AND CALCIUM FOR HEART HEALTH

Magnesium and calcium are important minerals with awesome but complementary roles in supporting cardiovascular fitness. Their significance may be summarized as follows:

1. Magnesium

Blood Pressure Regulation:

Vascular Health: Magnesium helps loosen up blood vessels, lowering vascular resistance and decreasing blood pressure. This is vital for stopping high blood pressure and decreasing the chance of cardiovascular ailment.

Electrolyte Balance: Magnesium aids in maintaining a right electrolyte stability, that is important for healthy blood pressure ranges.

Heart Rhythm and Function:

Arrhythmia Prevention: Adequate magnesium degrees help keep a regular coronary heart rhythm and save you arrhythmias (irregular heartbeats). Magnesium is important for the electric pastime of the coronary heart.

Muscle Relaxation: It supports the rest of smooth muscle mass, such as those inside the heart and blood vessels, which helps in preventing muscle cramps and spasms.

Overall Cardiovascular Health:

Anti Inflammatory Effects: Magnesium has anti inflammatory homes that can assist reduce persistent inflammation, a threat element for coronary heart sickness.

Cholesterol Levels: Some research endorse that magnesium may additionally impact levels of cholesterol, contributing to general cardiovascular health.

2. Calcium

Blood Pressure Regulation:

Vascular Function: Calcium is concerned inside the contraction and rest of blood vessels. Proper calcium degrees help hold ordinary blood vessel function and contribute to solid blood pressure.

Calcium Potassium Balance: Adequate calcium intake can help balance potassium levels, which additionally plays a position in blood stress regulation.

Heart Muscle Function:

Contraction: Calcium is vital for the contraction of heart muscle groups. It allows the heart to overcome successfully and preserve a normal rhythm.

CHAPTER 4: FOODS TO INCLUDE AND AVOID

BENEFICIAL FOODS

FRUITS AND VEGGIES

Fruits and Vegetables for Heart Health
Fruits and vegetables are essential components of a heart healthful food regimen, especially in the context of coping with blood pressure and basic cardiovascular health.

1. Benefits for Blood Pressure

High in Potassium:

Many end result and veggies are wealthy in potassium, which allows balance sodium tiers in the frame and loosen up blood vessels, for this reason decreasing blood strain.

Examples: Bananas, oranges, avocados, spinach, and sweet potatoes.

Low in Sodium:

Fruits and greens obviously comprise little to no sodium, making them an excellent choice for managing blood stress.

Examples: Fresh culmination (e.G., apples, berries) and vegetables (e.G., carrots, cucumbers).

2. Rich in Fiber

Digestive Health:

Fiber aids in digestion and helps alter blood sugar tiers, which is beneficial for cardiovascular fitness.

Examples: Beans, lentils, apples, and leafy veggies.

Cholesterol Management:

Soluble fiber observed in culmination and greens can assist lower LDL ldl cholesterol (bad cholesterol), that's critical for coronary heart fitness.

Examples: Oats, apples, and citrus fruits.

3. Antioxidants and Phytochemicals

Reduced Oxidative Stress:

Fruits and vegetables are rich in antioxidants, which assist reduce oxidative strain and irritation, both of which are linked to heart sickness.

Examples: Berries (e.G., blueberries, strawberries), tomatoes, and bell peppers.

Anti Inflammatory Properties:

Many culmination and vegetables comprise phytochemicals that have anti inflammatory consequences, that could assist defend the cardiovascular device.

Examples: Leafy greens (e.G., kale, spinach), and calciferous veggies (e.G., broccoli, Brussels sprouts).

4. Essential Vitamins and Minerals

Vitamin C:

Supports the health of blood vessels and helps lessen blood pressure.

Examples: Citrus culmination (e.G., oranges, grapefruits), strawberries, and kiwi.

Vitamin A:

Supports typical cardiovascular health and helps preserve healthy skin and tissues.

Examples: Carrots, candy potatoes, and dark leafy veggies.

Folate:

Important for reducing tiers of homocysteine, an amino acid linked to coronary heart ailment.

Examples: Spinach, broccoli, and oranges.

5. Practical Tips for Incorporating Fruits and Vegetables

Variety: Aim to encompass a huge range of colors and types to maximize nutrient intake and health blessings. Different shades regularly indicate one of a kind styles of antioxidants and vitamins.

Portion Size: Try to fill half of your plate with culmination and vegetables at each meal to make certain you're getting enough.

Snacking: Keep clean fruits and cutup greens handy for healthy snacks.

FOODS TO LIMIT OR AVOID FOR HEART HEALTH

To preserve highest quality heart fitness, in particular for managing blood stress and reducing the threat of cardiovascular sicknesses, it's vital to restriction or avoid certain foods.

1. High Sodium Foods

Processed Foods:

Examples: Canned soups, processed meats (e.G., bacon, sausages), and frozen dinners.

Reason: These ingredients often include excessive levels of delivered sodium, which could growth blood strain and contribute to fluid retention.

Salty Snacks:

Examples: Chips, pretzels, and salted nuts.

Reason: These snacks are excessive in sodium and might make contributions to excessive sodium consumption.

Restaurant and Fast Foods:

Examples: Burgers, fries, pizza, and fried meals.

Reason: Restaurant and fast meals objects are frequently excessive in sodium, dangerous fat, and added sugars.

2. Foods High in Saturated and Trans Fats

Red and Processed Meats:

Examples: Fatty cuts of pork, red meat, and processed meats like warm puppies and deli meats.

Reason: High in saturated fats, which could raise LDL (bad) cholesterol levels and make a contribution to heart sickness.

Fried Foods:

Examples: Fried chicken, French fries, and doughnuts.

Reason: Often cooked in oils high in trans fats, that can growth levels of cholesterol and promote inflammation.

Baked Goods:

Examples: Pastries, desserts, cookies, and certain margarine.

Reason: These merchandise often incorporate trans fats and excessive levels of introduced sugars and bad fats.

3. Added Sugars

Sugary Beverages:

Examples: Soda, sweetened coffee drinks, and energy liquids.

Reason: High in brought sugars, that may contribute to weight benefit, insulin resistance, and extended hazard of heart disorder.

Candy and Sweets:

Examples: Candy bars, goodies, and sugary desserts.

Reason: High in sugar and often mixed with unhealthy fats, contributing to poor coronary heart health.

High Sugar Breakfast Cereals:

Examples: Some flavored cereals and granola bars.

Reason: Often incorporate delivered sugars which could make contributions to high blood sugar ranges and poor basic heart health.

4. Excessive Alcohol

Impacts:

Reason: Drinking alcohol in excess can lead to high blood pressure, weight advantage, and accelerated chance of coronary heart ailment.

Guideline: If you consume alcohol, achieve this carefully—up to one drink in keeping with day for ladies and drinks in line with day for guys.

5. Foods High in Cholesterol

Egg Yolks:

Reason: High in dietary ldl cholesterol, that may contribute to multiplied blood cholesterol levels if ate up in extra.

Guideline: Limit intake and take into account the usage of egg whites or ldl cholesterol unfastened alternatives.

Certain Shellfish:

Examples: Shrimp and lobster.

Reason: While nutritious, some shellfish are excessive in ldl cholesterol. Moderation is key.

6. Highly Processed and Refined Foods

White Bread and Pasta:

Reason: Made from refined grains that are low in fiber and vitamins, which can make a contribution to terrible coronary heart health.

Alternative: Choose entire grain or entire wheat alternatives.

Instant Noodles and Rice:

Reason: Often high in sodium and lacking in crucial nutrients.

Alternative: Opt for whole grain variations and cook with clean substances.

TIPS FOR HEALTHIER CHOICES

Read Labels: Always check nutrition labels for sodium, fats, and sugar content.

Cook at Home: Prepare food using clean substances to control sodium, fats, and sugar content.

Choose Fresh: Opt for sparkling, unprocessed meals on every occasion possible.

SUGARY AND FATTY FOODS: IMPACT ON HEALTH AND HOW TO MANAGE

Sugary and fatty ingredients can notably have an effect on coronary heart health, blood pressure, and universal well being.

1. Sugary Foods

Impact on Health:

Weight Gain:

High Calorie Content: Sugary foods are often high in calories with little to no nutritional value, contributing to weight gain and weight problems.

Effect on Metabolism: Excessive sugar consumption can lead to insulin resistance and metabolic syndrome, increasing the threat of diabetes and heart sickness.

Increased Blood Pressure:

Fluid Retention: High sugar consumption can lead to fluid retention, which might also increase blood pressure.

Insulin Resistance: Excessive sugar can motive spikes in blood glucose degrees and affect blood strain law.

Dental Health:

Cavities and Decay: Sugars feed harmful micro organism inside the mouth, leading to tooth decay and gum sickness.

Common Sugary Foods to Limit:

Soda and Sweetened Beverages:

Examples: Regular sodas, sweetened iced teas, and strength beverages.

Candy and Sweets:

Examples: Candy bars, chocolate, pastries, and cookies.

Sweetened Breakfast Cereals:

Examples: Frosted cereals, granola bars with delivered sugars.

Desserts and Baked Goods:

Examples: Cakes, pies, doughnuts, and ice cream.

ALCOHOL AND CAFFEINE: IMPACT ON HEALTH AND GUIDELINES

Both acohol and caffeine can have an impact on numerous elements of health, consisting of blood pressure and cardiovascular fitness.

1. Alcohol

Impact on Health:

Blood Pressure:

Temporary Increase: Drinking alcohol can motive a temporary boom in blood strain.

Chronic Effects: Excessive alcohol consumption is associated with lengthy term high blood pressure and can exacerbate current high blood strain.

Heart Health:

Increased Risk: Heavy alcohol use can cause cardiomyopathy (a condition wherein the coronary heart muscle weakens), arrhythmias, and a higher risk of heart disease.

Weight Gain: Alcohol is excessive in empty energy, that could make a contribution to weight gain and weight problems, in addition affecting cardiovascular health.

Liver Health:

Alcoholic Liver Disease: Excessive ingesting can result in liver infection, fatty liver disease, and cirrhosis.

Guidelines for Consumption:

Moderation: The American Heart Association recommends restricting alcohol intake to:

Women: Up to one drink according to day.

Men: Up to 2 liquids in keeping with day.

Definition of a Standard Drink:

Beer: 12 oz. (355 ml).

Wine: 5 ounces (148 ml).

Spirits: 1.5 oz (forty four ml).

Tips for Managing Alcohol Intake:

Track Consumption: Keep a record of ways a lot you drink to make certain you stay inside advocated limits.

Choose Lower Alcohol Options: Opt for liquids with decrease alcohol content and drink slowly.

Avoid Binge Drinking: Limit the frequency of heavy ingesting periods.

2. Caffeine

Impact on Health:

Blood Pressure:

Short Term Increase: Caffeine can purpose a temporary spike in blood strain due to its stimulating results on the cardiovascular machine.

Long Term Effects: While slight caffeine consumption isn't always generally related to sustained excessive blood strain, immoderate intake can make a contribution to hypertension in susceptible people.

Heart Health:

Arrhythmia: High doses of caffeine can lead to palpitations or irregular heartbeats in touchy people.

Bone Health: Excessive caffeine intake can affect calcium absorption, probably impacting bone health.

Sleep and Anxiety:

Disrupted Sleep: Caffeine can interfere with sleep patterns and cause insomnia if consumed too past due within the day.

Increased Anxiety: High caffeine intake can contribute to feelings of anxiety and jitteriness.

Guidelines for Consumption:

Moderation: Most health corporations propose maintaining caffeine consumption to approximately four hundred mg consistent with day, that's roughly equal to four 8ounce cups of brewed coffee.

Sensitive Individuals: Some humans may want to consume much less caffeine because of personal sensitivity or present health situations.

CHAPTER 5: MONITORING AND ADJUSTING YOUR DIET

TRACKING YOUR PROGRESS

TOOLS FOR MONITORING BLOOD PRESSURE

Monitoring blood strain is critical for handling high blood pressure and preserving cardiovascular fitness. There are several gear available, ranging from domestic devices to expert equipment.

1. Digital Blood Pressure Monitors

Automatic Upper Arm Monitors:

Description: These gadgets inflate mechanically and offer a virtual readout of blood stress and pulse price. They are normally accurate and easy to use.

Advantages: Convenient, person friendly, and typically offers accurate readings.

Examples: Omron, Withings, and Beurer.

Wrist Monitors:

Description: These devices degree blood stress on the wrist. They are transportable and easy to use but can be less accurate than higher arm video display units if no longer positioned efficiently.

Advantages: Compact and portable.

Examples: Omron, iHealth, and Greater Goods.

Finger Monitors:

Description: These gadgets measure blood strain using a finger cuff. They are less generally used due to concerns about accuracy.

Advantages: Portable and smooth to use.

Examples: Some models are available from manufacturers like Veridian.

Examples: Classic brands consist of Welch Allyn and ADC.

2. Ambulatory Blood Pressure Monitors
24Hour Monitoring Devices:

Description: These gadgets are worn for 24 hours to record blood pressure at normal intervals at some point of the day and night.

Advantages: Provides a comprehensive view of blood pressure variations through the years and enables diagnose conditions like white coat hypertension.

Examples: Available via healthcare providers and specialized clinical gadget providers.

3. Smartphone Apps and Wearable Devices
Blood Pressure Apps:

Description: Apps that work in conjunction with outside video display units to track and file blood pressure readings.

Advantages: Allows for easy tracking and analysis of trends over time.

Examples: Apps like Omron Connect and Withing Health Mate.

Wearable Devices:

Description: Some health trackers and smartwatches have integrated blood stress monitoring features.

Advantages: Provides continuous monitoring and integrates with different health metrics.

Examples: Some fashions from Fitbit, Apple Watch, and Garmin offer blood pressure monitoring features.

4. Home Monitoring Kits

Complete Kits:

Description: These kits regularly encompass a blood strain display, stethoscope, and different accessories for comprehensive monitoring.

Advantages: Provides a whole solution for domestic monitoring.

Examples: Kits from brands like Omron and Withings.

ADAPTING YOUR DIET AS NEEDED

Adapting your eating regimen is a crucial step in dealing with excessive blood pressure and selling ordinary health.

1. Assess Your Current Diet

Track Your Intake: Keep a meals diary to monitor what you're ingesting, inclusive of quantities and frequency. This helps perceive styles and areas for improvement.

Evaluate Nutritional Content: Review the dietary content material of your modern day weight loss plan, specializing in sodium, sugar, fats, and universal calorie intake.

2. Focus on Key Nutrients

Increase PotassiumRich Foods:

Benefits: Potassium enables stability sodium levels and supports healthy blood strain.

Examples: Bananas, oranges, potatoes, and leafy greens.

Boost Magnesium and Calcium Intake:

Benefits: Both minerals guide coronary heart health and blood pressure law.

Examples: Magnesiumrich meals consist of nuts, seeds, and whole grains. Calciumrich meals consist of dairy merchandise and fortified plant primarily based milks.

Limit Sodium Intake:

Strategy: Reduce or dispose of high sodium ingredients and use herbs and spices for flavoring in preference to salt.

Examples: Opt for clean meals over processed objects and examine labels for sodium content.

Moderate Saturated and Trans Fats:

Strategy: Choose more healthy fats, along with the ones discovered in avocados, nuts, and olive oil, and restriction consumption of fried and processed meals.

Examples: Replace fatty meats with lean proteins and pick out complete grain merchandise over refined alternatives.

Reduce Added Sugars:

Strategy: Limit sugary snacks and beverages. Opt for natural sources of sweetness, like culmination.

Examples: Avoid sugary drinks and select entire fruits over fruit juices.

3. Personalize Your Diet

Consider Health Conditions: Adapt your weight reduction plan based on any extra health conditions, which includes diabetes or kidney sickness, which could require specific dietary modifications.

Monitor Blood Pressure Regularly: Track how dietary adjustments affect your blood strain over time and modify as wished.

Consult a Dietitian: A registered dietitian can offer customized recommendation and meal making plans primarily based for your precise desires and fitness goals.

4. Incorporate Healthy Eating Habits

Balanced Meals: Ensure each meal consists of a combination of fruits, veggies, whole grains, lean proteins, and healthy fat.

Portion Control: Be aware of element sizes to avoid overeating and manage weight.

Stay Hydrated: Drink masses of water throughout the day to support typical fitness and assist adjust blood pressure.

Meal Planning: Plan meals beforehand to make sure you have got wholesome options available and decrease reliance on convenience meals.

5. Adapt to Lifestyle Changes

Physical Activity: Combine dietary changes with everyday physical interest to decorate standard health and help blood stress management.

Stress Management: Incorporate stress decreasing strategies, together with mindfulness or yoga, as pressure can impact blood strain and consuming conduct.

Regular Checkups: Regular visits in your healthcare company can help reveal progress and make essential nutritional modifications.

6. Example Meal Adjustments

Breakfast: Replace sugary cereals with oatmeal crowned with fresh fruit and nuts.

Lunch: Choose a salad with lots of colorful veggies, a lean protein source (like grilled chicken), and a light French dressing.

Dinner: Opt for baked fish or a plant based protein with a aspect of steamed vegetables and quinoa.

Snacks: Select uncooked vegetables with hummus or a piece of fruit with a handful of nuts.

WHEN TO SEEK PROFESSIONAL HELP

Seeking professional assistance is essential if you have concerns approximately your blood pressure or in case you revel in signs associated with cardiovascular fitness.

1. Persistent High Blood Pressure

Consistently Elevated Readings: If your blood stress readings are consistently above the everyday variety (120/eighty mmHg) regardless of making way of life modifications, it's important to seek advice from a healthcare provider.

Frequent Monitoring: If you're continuously getting high readings at domestic or from a monitoring tool, searching for professional evaluation to decide the motive and appropriate remedy.

2. Symptoms of Hypertension

Headaches and Dizziness: Frequent or severe complications, dizziness, or lightheartedness may be symptoms of excessive blood pressure or different health issues.

Chest Pain: Experiencing chest pain or soreness could imply a serious circumstance, along with heart disorder or a heart assault.

Shortness of Breath: Difficulty respiration or shortness of breath, in particular if followed with the aid of other signs and symptoms, have to be evaluated promptly.

3. Risk Factors or Existing Conditions

Family History: If you've got a family records of high blood pressure, heart disorder, or stroke, normal monitoring and expert consultation are critical.

Diabetes: People with diabetes need to manipulate their blood pressure carefully to keep away from headaches. If you have got diabetes, searching for expert help for tailored control techniques.

Kidney Disease: High blood stress can affect kidney characteristic, so if you have kidney disorder, everyday check united states with a healthcare company are important.

4. Difficulty Managing Lifestyle Changes

Struggling with Diet and Exercise: If you locate it challenging to make or hold nutritional and way of life modifications, a healthcare issuer or dietitian can offer personalized steerage and support.

Medication Management: If you're having hassle adhering to prescribed medications or experiencing facet results, seek advice from your healthcare provider for changes or options.

5. Unexplained Symptoms or Concerns

New or Unusual Symptoms: If you experience new or unexplained signs and symptoms, consisting of swelling, imaginative and prescient changes, or uncommon fatigue, are seeking expert assessment.

Concerns About Blood Pressure Medications: If you've got concerns or questions about your blood stress medications, consisting of their effectiveness or facet consequences, discuss them along with your healthcare company.

6. Follow Up and Regular Check Ups

Routine Monitoring: Regular observe up appointments with your healthcare issuer are important to screen your blood pressure and adjust treatment as needed.

Periodic Testing: Regular blood exams and reviews can be necessary to test for headaches or to evaluate the effectiveness of remedy.

WHEN TO SEEK IMMEDIATE HELP

Emergency Symptoms: If you experience extreme signs inclusive of unexpected chest pain, trouble breathing, excessive headache, or signs and symptoms of a stroke (e.G., sudden numbness, confusion, hassle speaking), seek emergency medical assist without delay.

MAKING ADJUSTMENTS BASED ON FEEDBACK

Adapting and enhancing your method to handling blood pressure often requires making modifications based on comments from various sources.

1. Feedback from Medical Professionals

Follow Up Appointments:

Review Results: Discuss the results of blood stress readings and any assessments with your healthcare issuer. Understand how these consequences replicate your health popularity and treatment efficacy.

Adjust Treatment: If your cutting edge plan isn't running in addition to expected, your company may endorse modifications in remedy, weight loss program, or lifestyle.

Medication Reviews:

Assess Side Effects: If you enjoy aspect results from medication, inform your healthcare company. They may also adjust the dosage or switch to a one of a kind medicine.

Effectiveness: Discuss how nicely the medicine is controlling your blood stress and any new signs and symptoms that arise.

2. Personal Monitoring Feedback

Track Your Progress:

Daily Readings: Regularly monitor your blood pressure at home and preserve a log of the readings. Note any patterns or changes based totally on nutritional or way of life adjustments.

Assess Trends: Look for tendencies to your readings to determine if adjustments are having the favored effect.

Diet and Exercise Logs:

Dietary Adjustments: If you've made modifications in your weight reduction plan (e.G., reducing sodium or increasing potassium), music how these changes effect your blood pressure.

Exercise Impact: Record your physical hobby and its effects to your blood stress and overall fitness.

3. Lifestyle Feedback

Evaluate Lifestyle Changes:

Dietary Impact: Assess how new nutritional conduct are affecting your blood pressure. Adjust your food regimen based totally on whether you're seeing wonderful or terrible modifications.

Exercise Routine: Monitor how ordinary physical activity impacts your blood strain and standard nicely being. Modify your exercise routine primarily based on what works pleasant for you.

Stress and Sleep:

Monitor Stress Levels: Track how stress management strategies are impacting your blood pressure. Adjust your strain reduction strategies if necessary.

Evaluate Sleep Quality: Assess the effect of your sleep styles on your blood pressure. Make adjustments to enhance sleep if wanted.

4. Personal Feedback and Observations

Listen to Your Body:

Symptom Monitoring: Pay attention to any new or changing symptoms. Use this feedback to modify your fitness management techniques.

Self Assessment: Reflect on how properly your current techniques are operating. If you're now not seeing the anticipated consequences, remember editing your method.

Behavioral Adjustments:

Habit Changes: If sure behavior aren't helping your blood strain desires, make changes. For instance, if snacking on high sodium meals is a assignment, locate healthier alternatives.

5. Use Technology and Apps

Review App Data:

Track Patterns: Utilize health apps to song your blood strain, diet, and interest. Review app generated insights to make informed modifications.

Set Goals: Use apps to set and song desires, and adjust based on the feedback provided by using the app.

www.ingramcontent.com/pod-product-compliance
Lightning Source LLC
Chambersburg PA
CBHW072052230526
45479CB00010B/846